BALD

IS

BEAUTIFUL

TOO

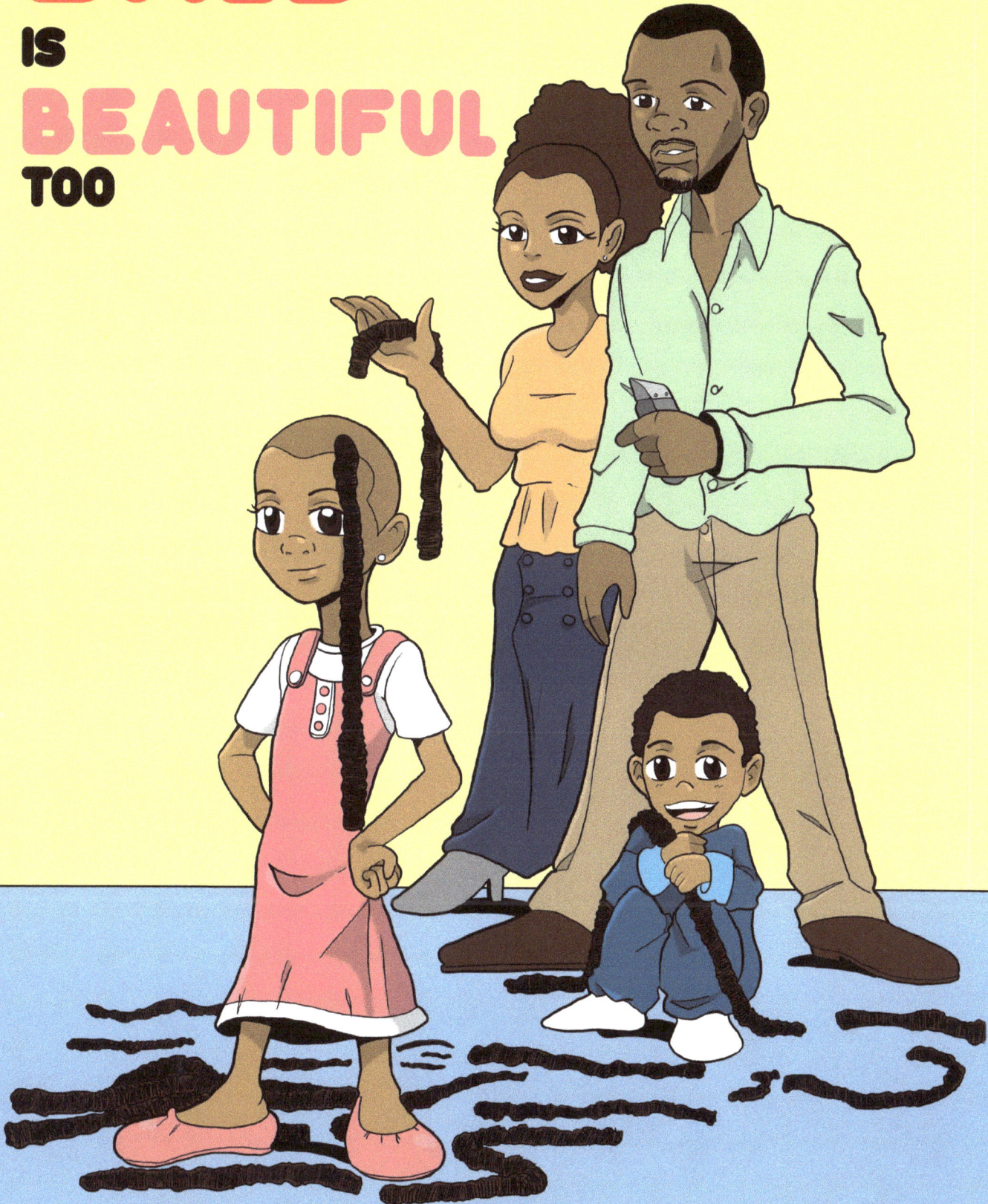

Monica Beasley-Martin

Copyright © 2013 by Monica Beasley– Martin

Printed in USA by Greater Is He Publishing

Editor: Shann Hall-Lochmann Van Bennekom

Illustrations: Eric Nyamor

Layout & Design: Ileta Randall

ISBN 978-1-938950-43-6

Greater is He Publishing

9824 E. Washington St. Chagrin Falls Ohio 44023

P O. Box 46115 Bedford Ohio, 44146

http://www.greaterishepublishing.com

216-288-9315

DEDICATION

Dedicated to my godson, Bryant Williams, who won his battle against cancer, and granddaughters, Janiah Beasley-Williams, who was the first to call me a bald head at the encouragement of big sister, Daja Beasley-Williams.

ABOUT THE AUTHOR

Diagnosed with alopecia in her twenties, Monica Beasley-Martin successfully hid her bald spots until 2006. Around this time, her godson began to lose his waist-long dreads from cancer treatments. In solidarity with him, Monica had her own remaining hair removed. This prompted her toddler granddaughter (encouraged by her older sister) to call her a bald head. Monica would hear this name repeated, often by the students in schools where she works as a substitute teacher. The taunts of these children inspired her to write, *"Bald is Beautiful, Too."* Monica, who is also an ordained minister and a drama teacher, lives in Youngstown, Ohio, with her husband, son, and dog, Soda Pop.

Nia Nefertiti Jones was eight years old with caramel-colored skin and waist-length dreadlocks. Everywhere Nia went, folks talked about her beautiful hair.

Miss Scott, who was more like an auntie than a neighbor, lived in the lemon-colored house next door. She always greeted Nia by saying hello in Swahili. When Nia walked by, Miss Scott waved and said, "Jambo!"

Nia smiled and answered, "Jambo, Miss Scott!"

Miss Scott chuckled. "Child you are a sight for sore eyes, you and all that pretty long hair."

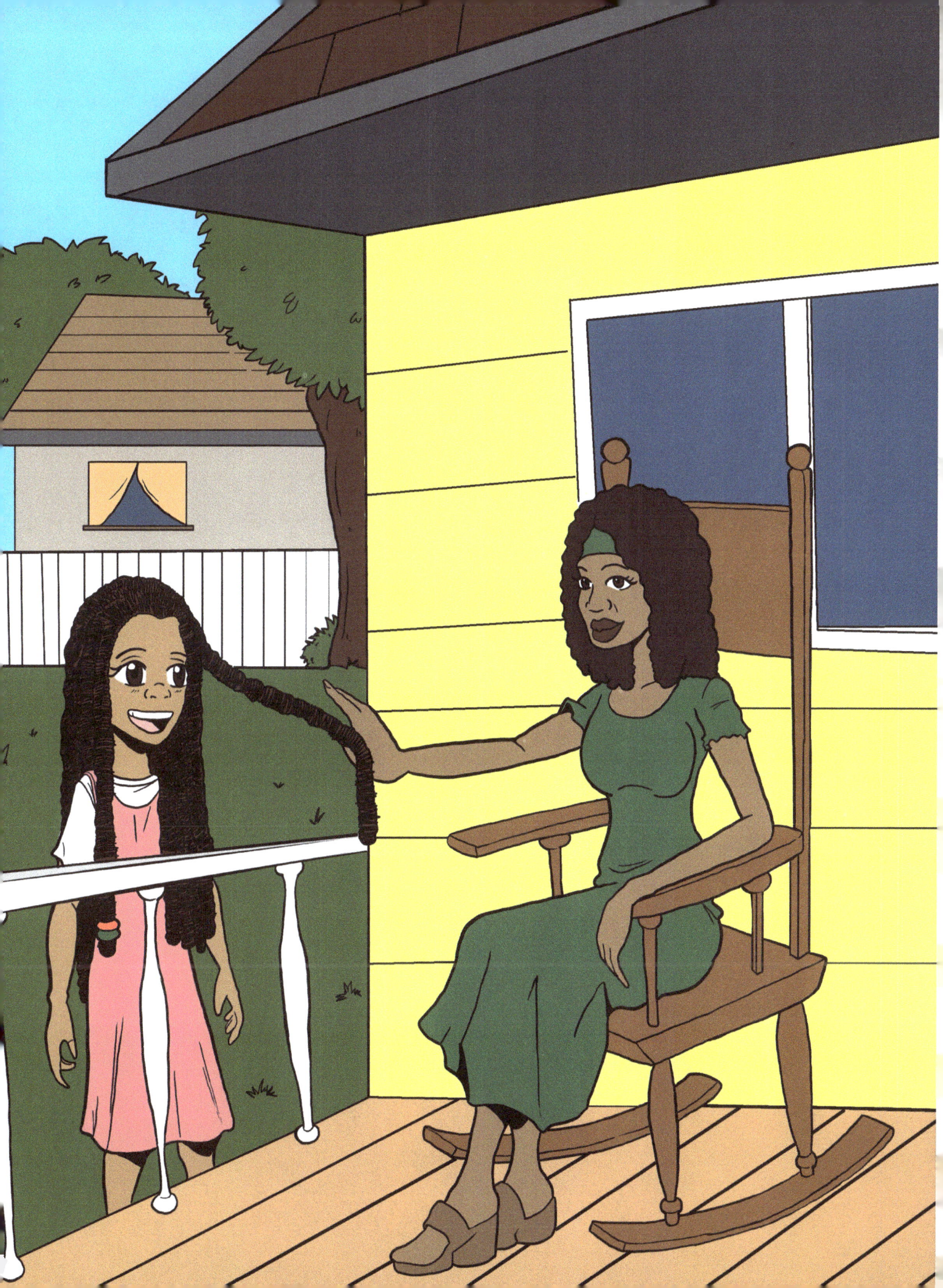

Nia's baby brother, Ode, loved to pretend that his sister's hair was a tent. Nia and Ode would make up stories. Ode would duck under Nia's hair to hide from pretend monsters. Nia's hair kept him safe.

Momma and Daddy laughed as they watched them. They loved their children very much. It made them happy to see Nia and Ode play together.

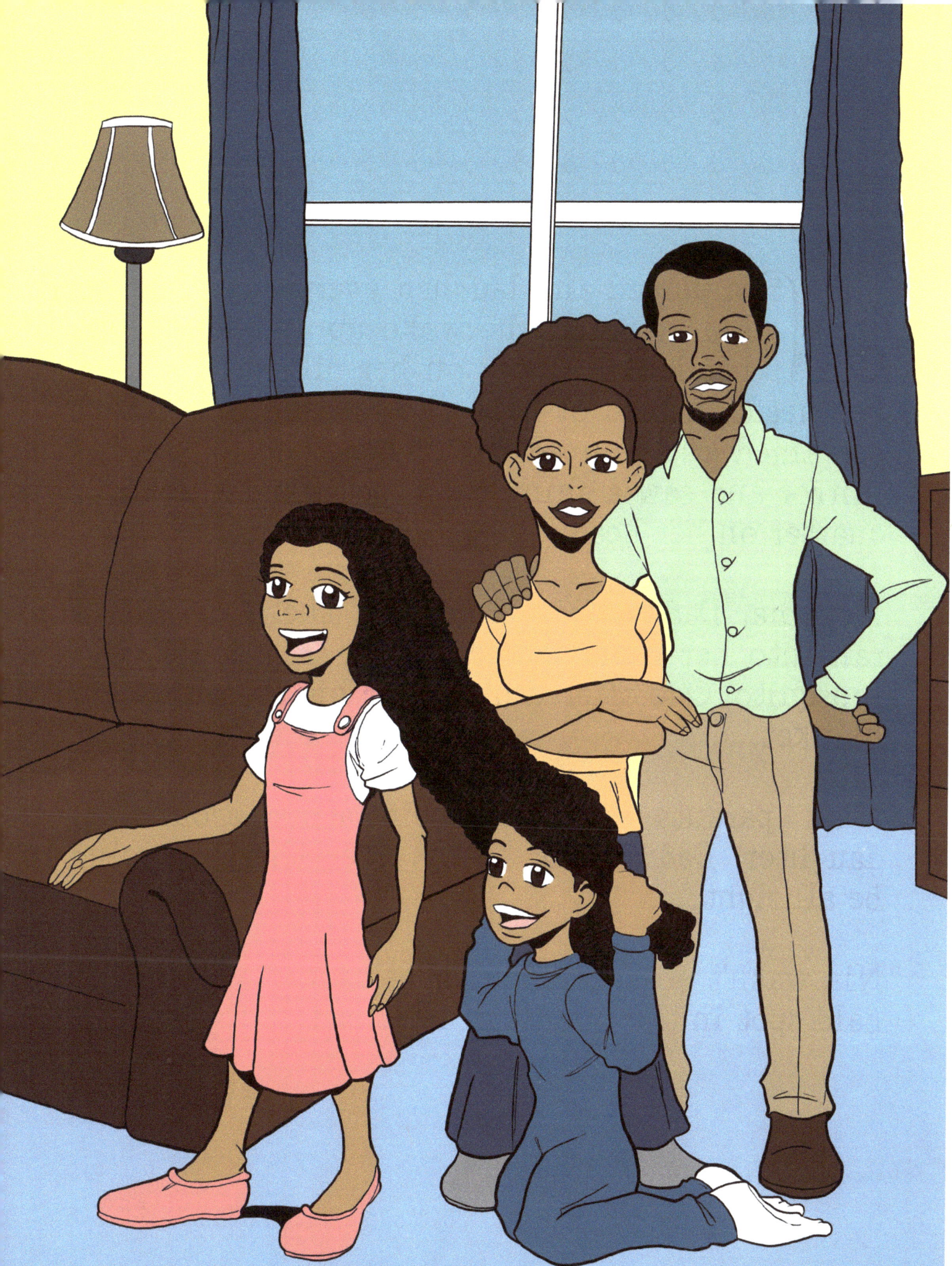

Nia played and laughed every day. One horrible morning she woke up and found one of her locks lying on her pillow. Nia touched her head. Instead of hair, she felt smooth skin. Nia screamed and jumped out of bed. She looked in the mirror and saw a shiny bald spot about the size of a quarter on her head.

Momma, Daddy, Ode, and even the dog, Soda Pop, ran into her room faster than a frog could catch a mosquito. Ode offered his sister his favorite security blanket.

Nia's parents wrapped their arms around their daughter. Daddy said, "Baby, everything is going to be all right."

Nia wasn't so sure about that. After all, she had a bald spot in the middle of her head.

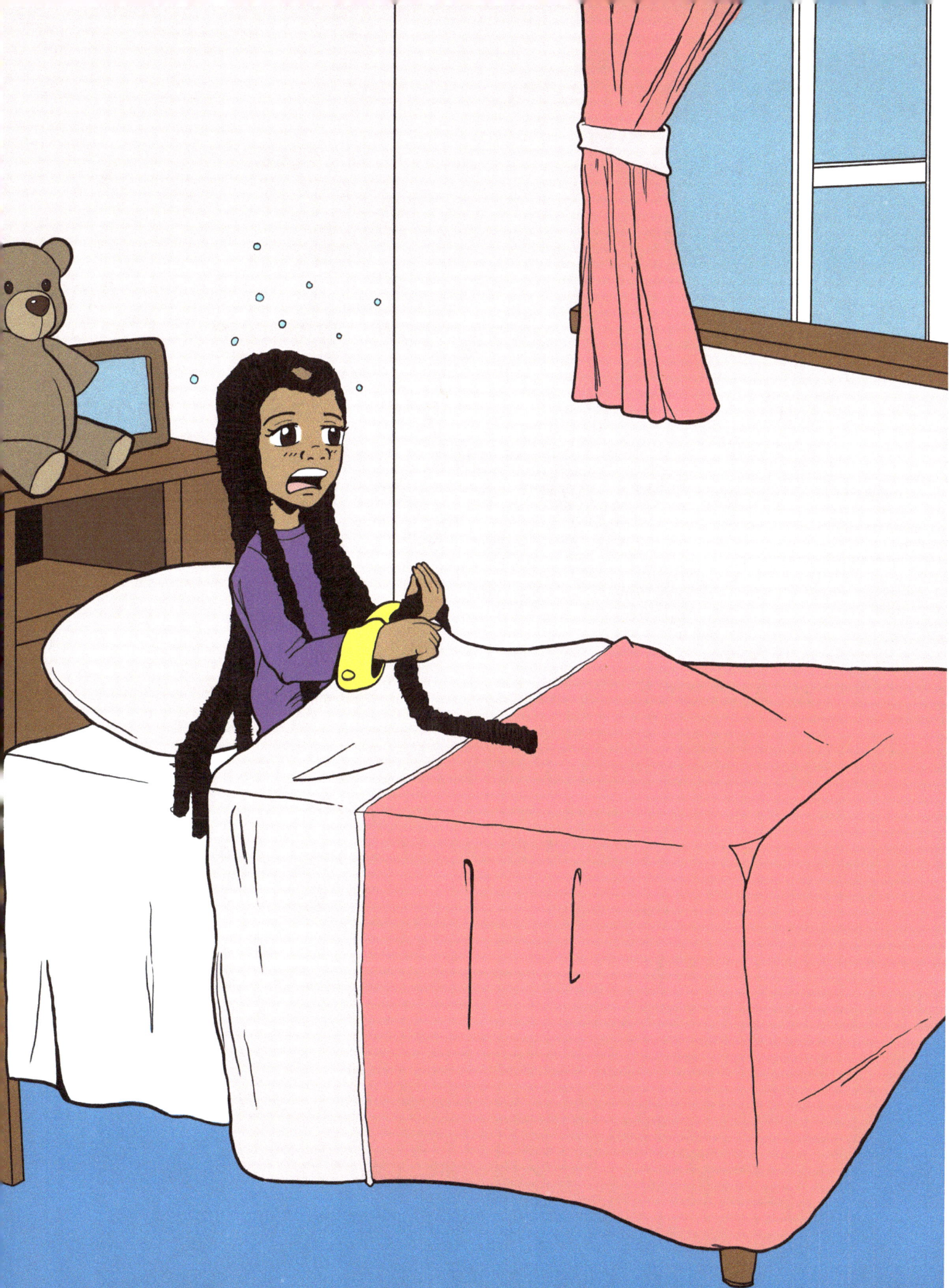

The next day, Nia's parents took her to see a dermatologist. Dr. Jada Brown was one of the best skin doctors in the city. After the doctor examined Nia, she said, "Nia has a condition known as alopecia. That's a fancy way of saying you're kind of allergic to your hair. Your body thinks that your hair is something bad, so it's trying to get rid of it. That's why your hair fell out."

Nia's eyes filled with tears as she looked at Dr. Brown and said, "Will it grow back?"

Doctor Brown replied, "It's hard to say. Sometimes it will grow back, but you also might lose more hair. Only time will tell." She patted Nia on the shoulder and smiled.

Nia looked into the doctor's sparkling eyes and managed to smile back.

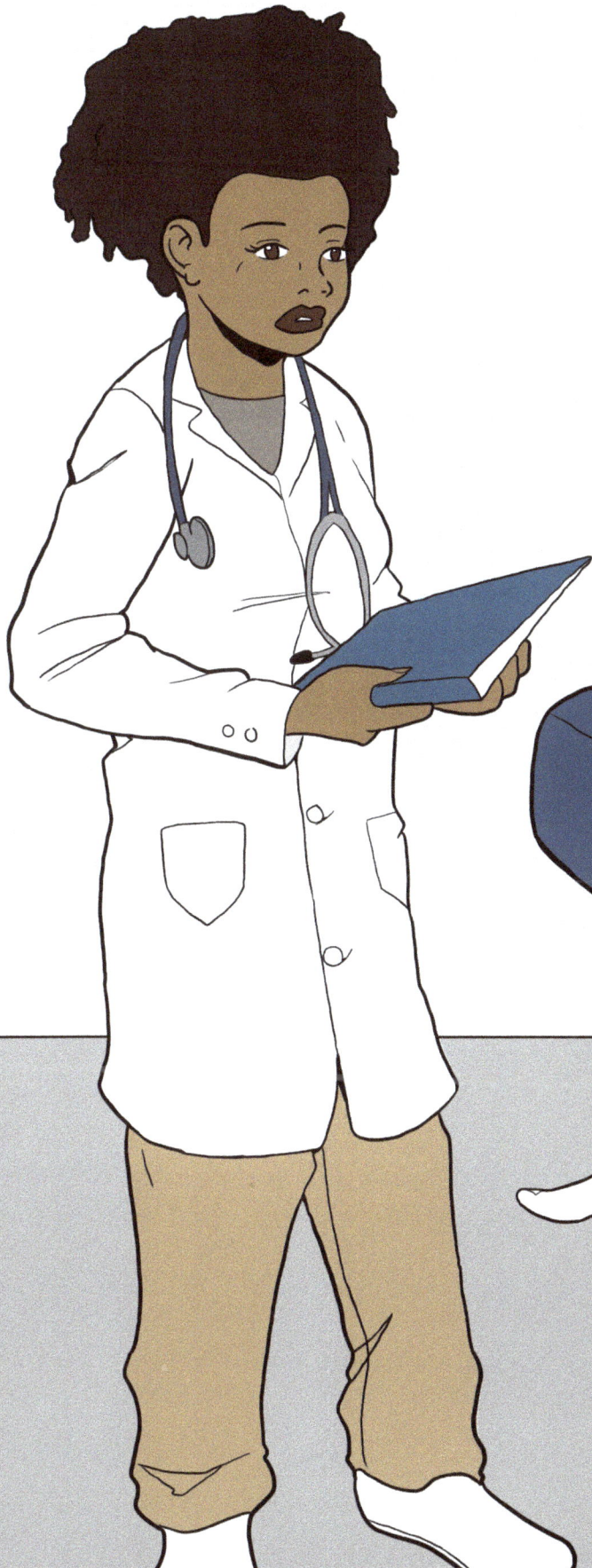

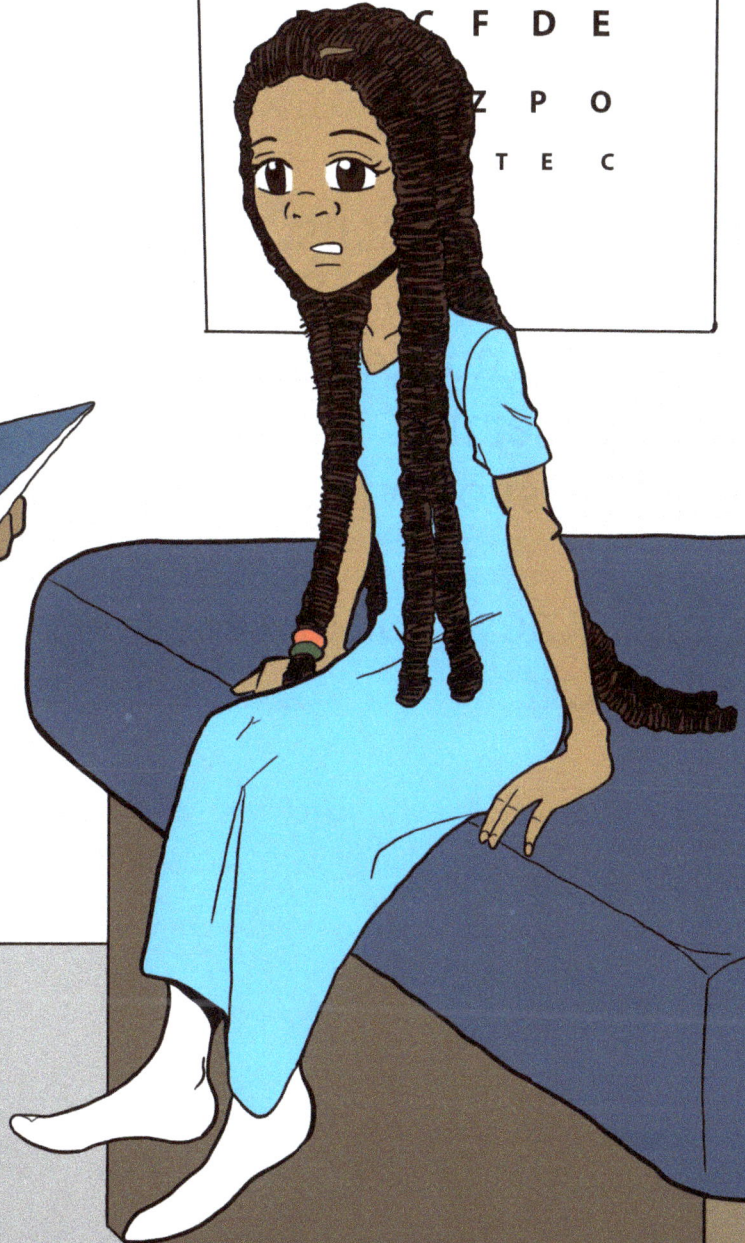

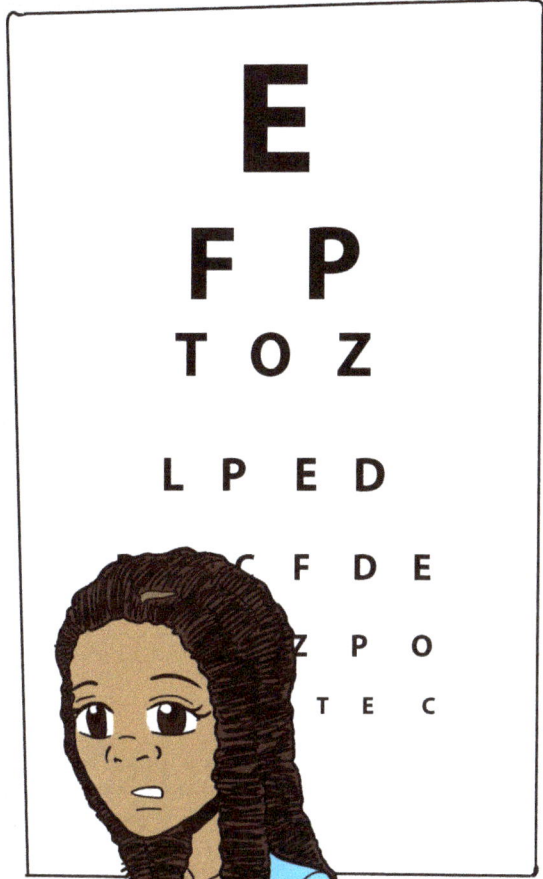

Dr. Brown gave Nia a sticker.

She mumbled, "Thank you." Then she and her parents went back home.

For several months, Momma did an excellent job of hiding that spot. She would pull Nia's hair up into a ponytail. Another time she'd wrap it with a colorful kente-patterned cloth scarf. Sometimes she would cover the spot with a pretty headband.

No one knew could tell that Nia had a bald spot on her head.

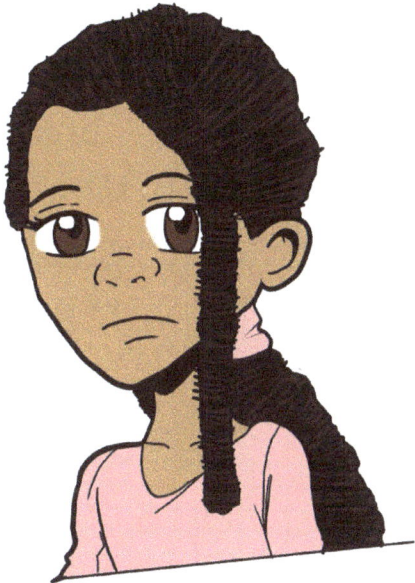

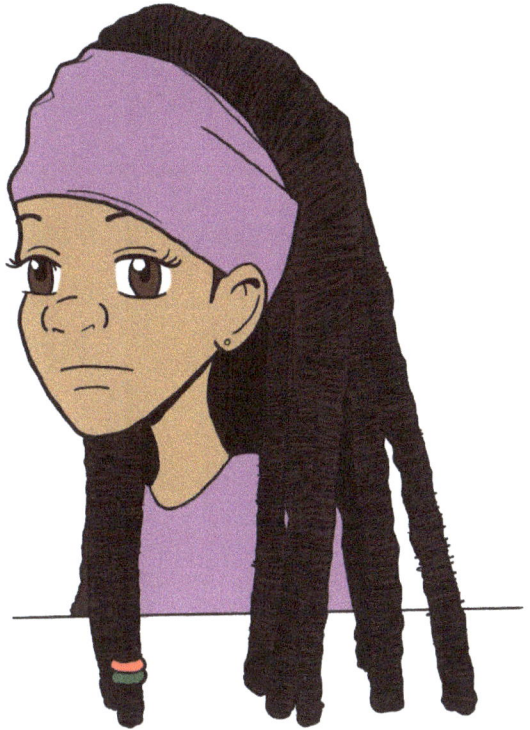

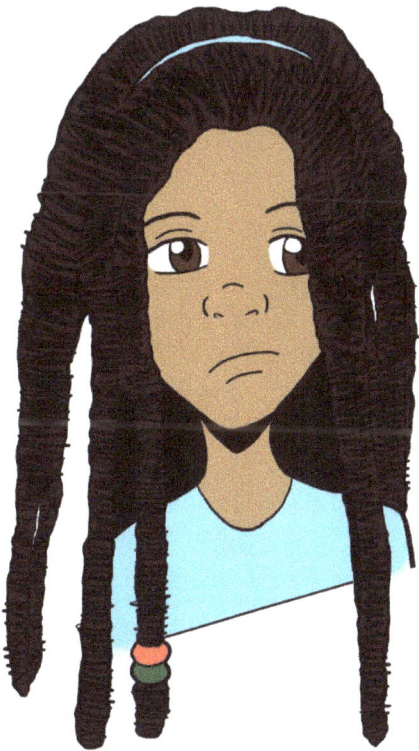

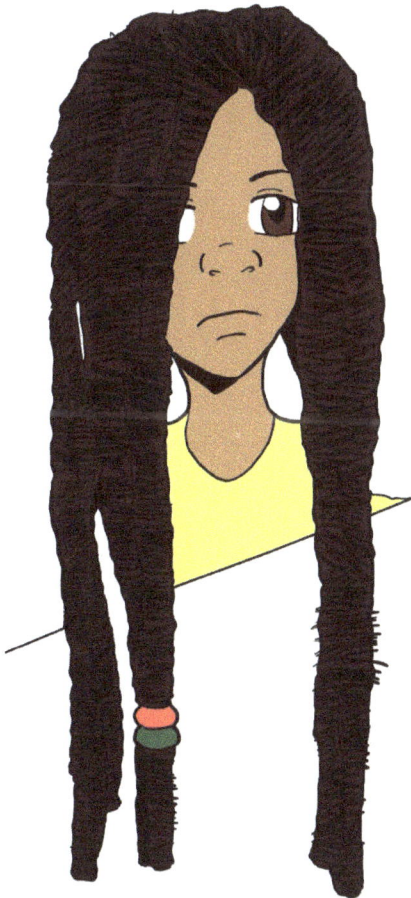

One day after school, Nia was walking down the hall. Her long hair was swinging back and forth. Suddenly, several more dreads fell off her head, like the flight of autumn leaves from trees just before winter.

Several boys playing nearby spotted Nia's hair on the ground. One boy pointed his finger and yelled, "She's a bald head! Nia's a bald head! Nia's a bald head!"

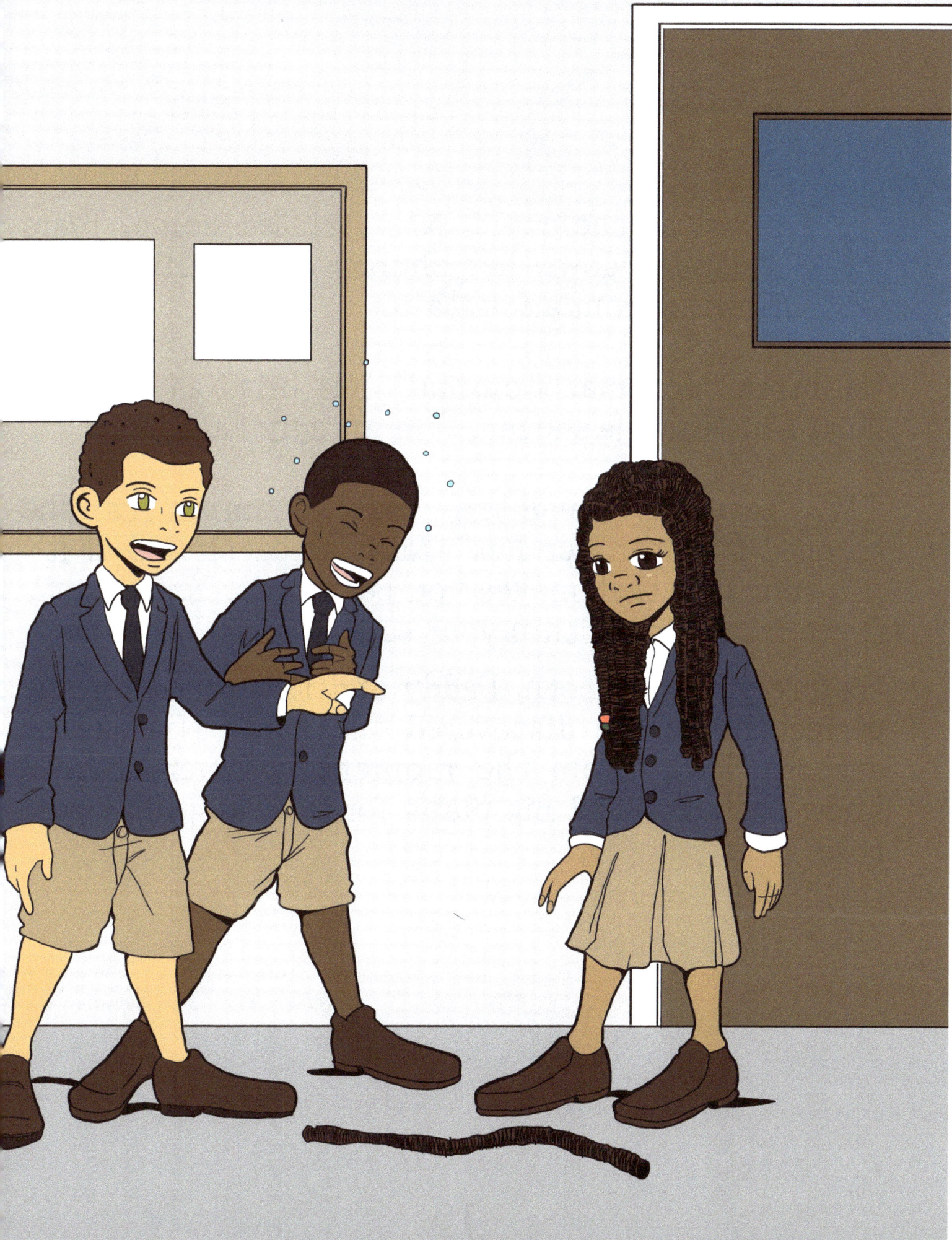

As fast as she could, Nia sprinted home. Tears streamed down her chubby cheeks like water flowing from a fountain.

"Momma, Momma, Momma!" Nia cried as she collapsed in Momma's arms. "I'm an ugly bald head!"

"My beautiful daughter, "said Momma as she scooped Nia into her lap." Bald is beautiful too! It's not your hair that makes you beautiful. Your beauty flows from deep within your soul.

"Before you were born, Daddy and I searched for the perfect name. We discovered the name Nia means purpose. Right from the moment you were born I knew that God had big plans for you, a special purpose."

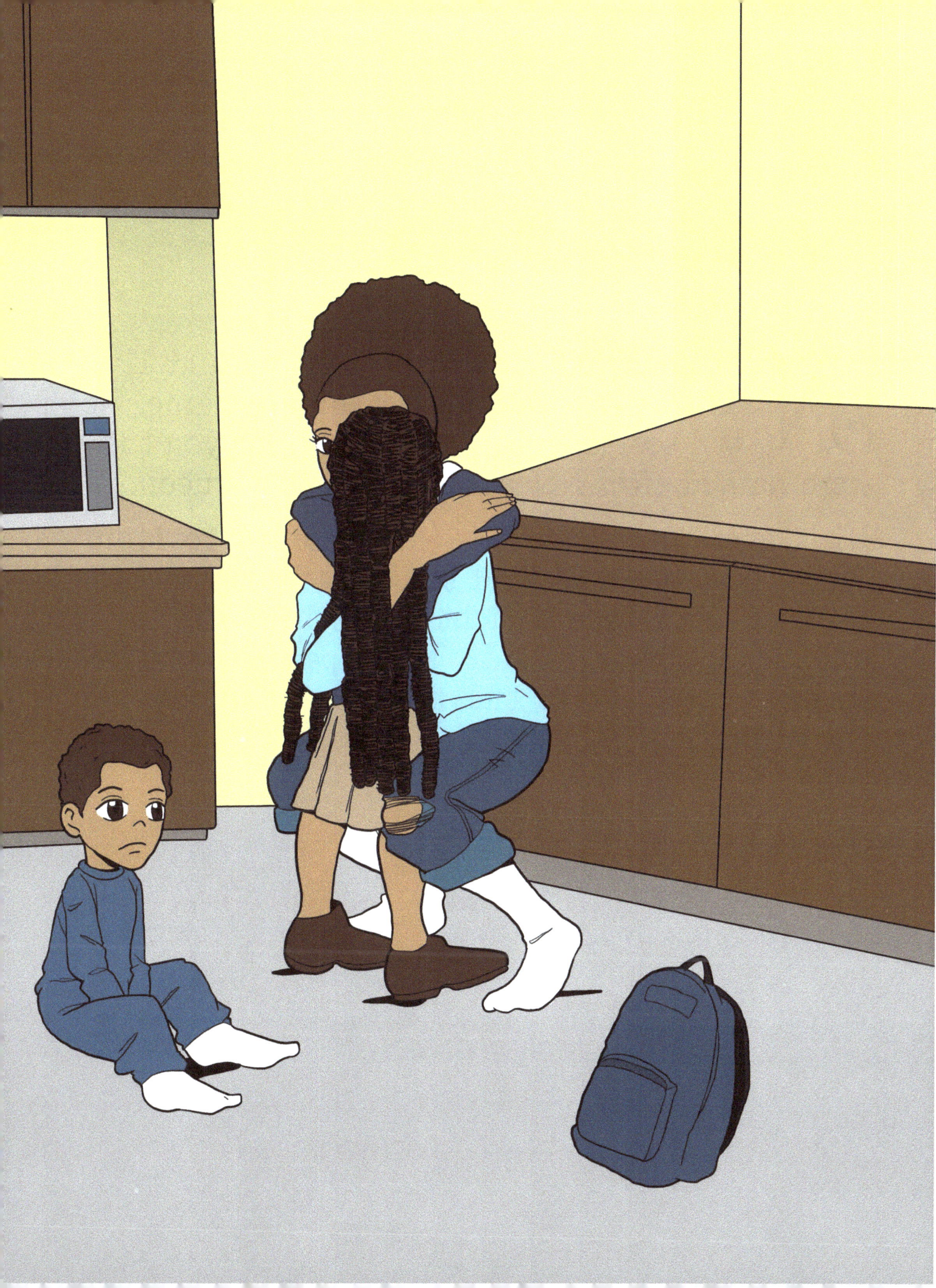

Nia snuggled closer to Momma and listened as Momma said, "Your middle name, Nefertiti seems to be a perfect fit for you too. You were named after Nefertiti, the African queen."

Nia's eyes grew bigger as she listened to Momma. "You know, she was bald too." Momma touched the back of Nia's head. "Right about here she had just one single strand of hair. Many people consider her to have been one of the most beautiful women in the world."

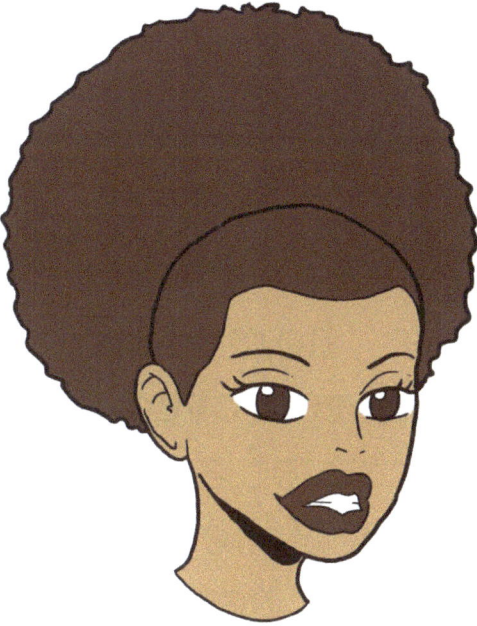

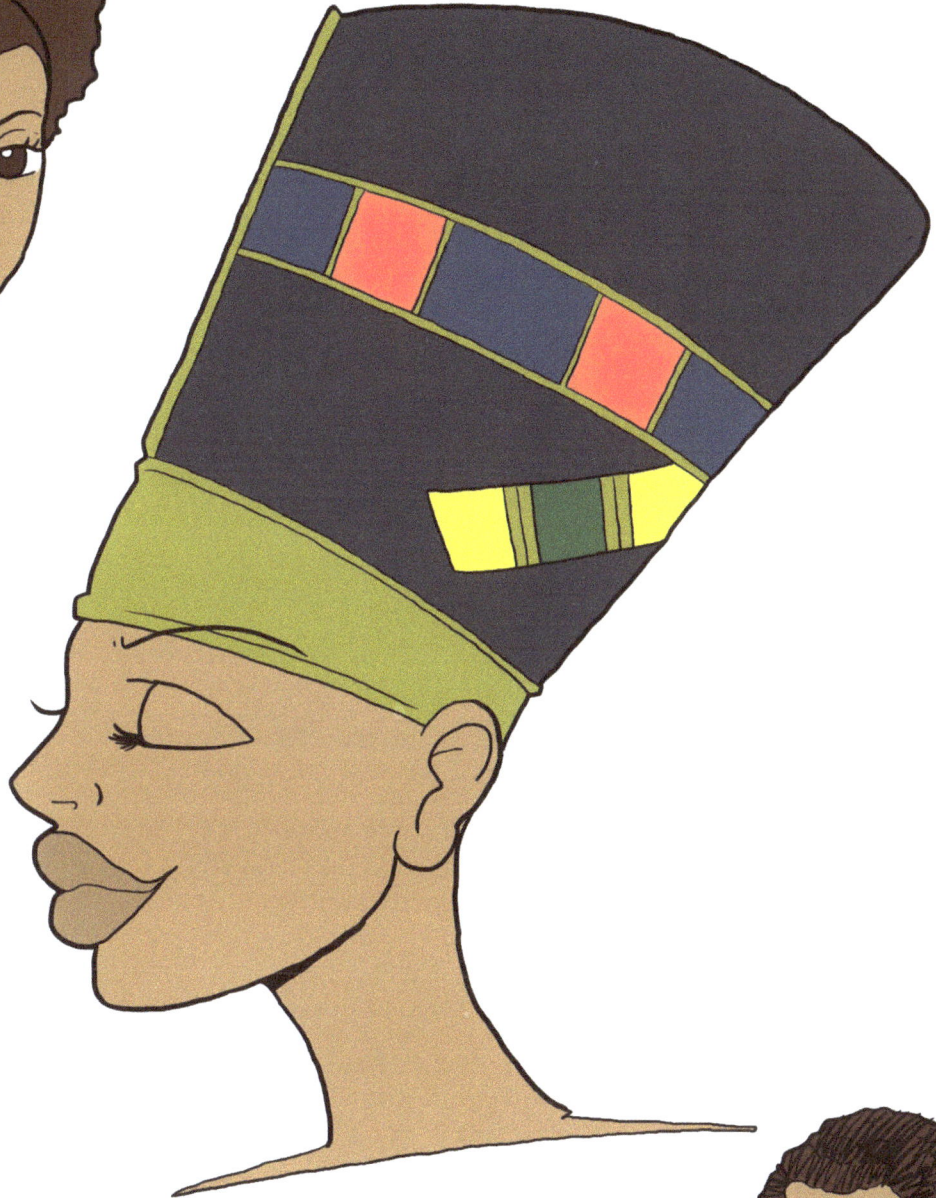

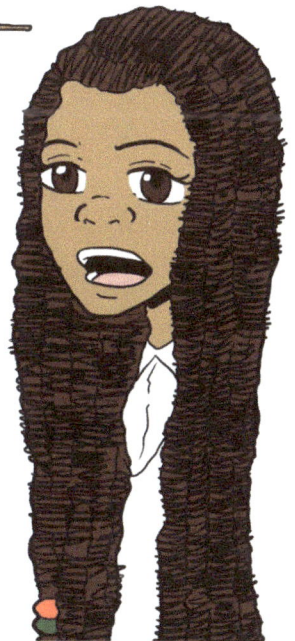

Later that evening, Daddy came home from work. He took out his clippers and removed the rest of Nia's hair-with the exception of a single lock at the back of her head. The next time somebody had the nerve to call her a bald head, Nia proudly announced, "Yes, I am! Bald is beautiful too. Let me tell you about Queen Nefertiti."

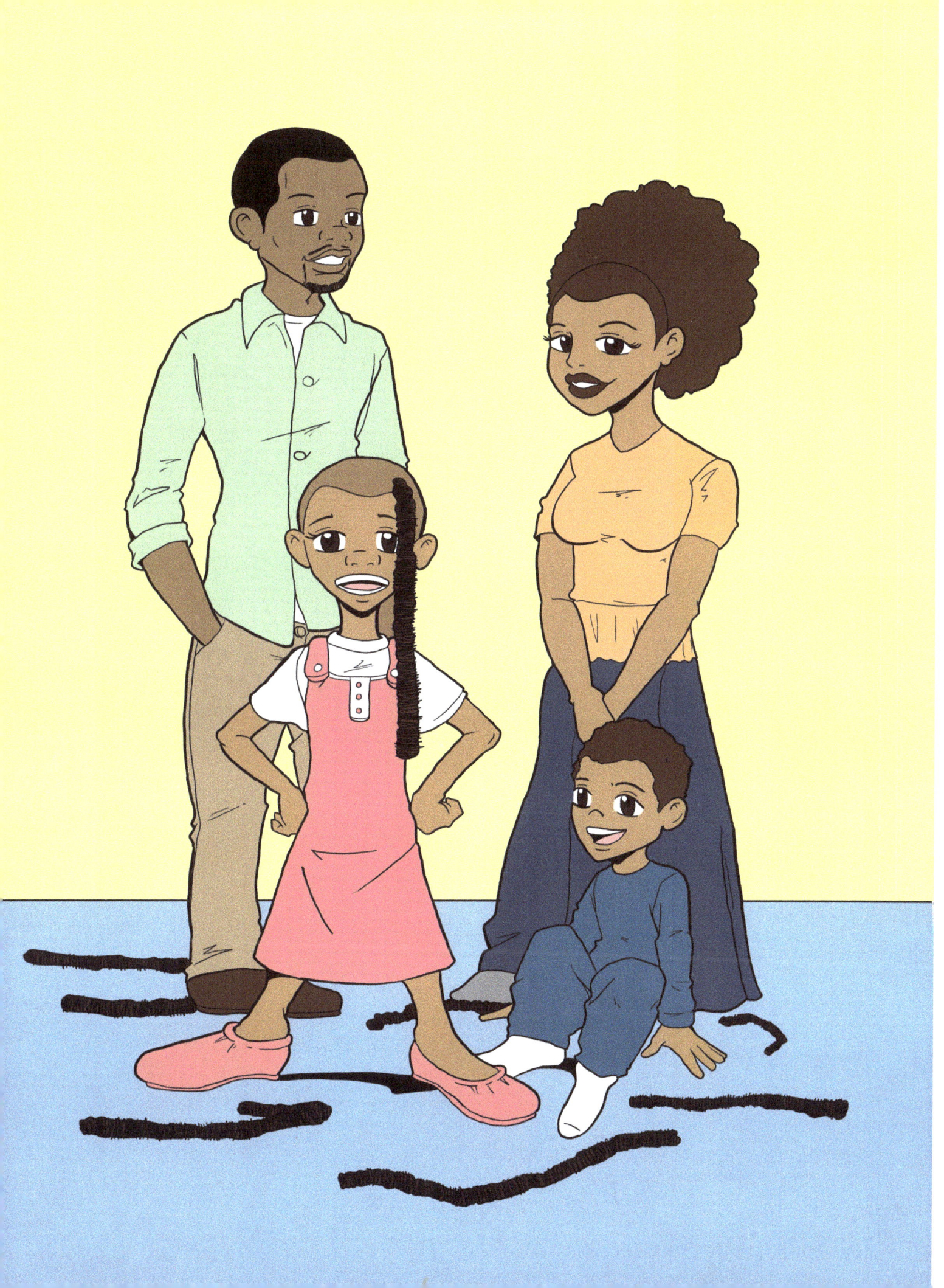